Written and Designed by Andrea Bonhiver

Copyright © 2019 Andrea Bonhiver.
All rights reserved. This book may not be reproduced in any form, in whole or in part (beyond the copying permitted by the US Copyright Law, Section 107, "fair use" in teaching research, Section 108, certain library copying, or in published media by reviews in limited excerpts), without written notarized permission from the author, Andrea Bonhiver.

Disclaimer
This book is for educational and enrichment purposes only. The views expressed are those of the author alone. The reader is responsible for his or her own actions. Neither the author nor the publisher assumes any responsibility or liability whatsoever on the behalf of the purchaser or reader of these materials.

this will not define you

(but it will change you.)

so, i guess this is real.

Those are the first words I wrote on the blank page that would become my lifeline throughout my cancer journey. In the span of a ten-minute phone call, I'd learned that not only did I have cervical cancer, but I would soon need a hysterectomy that would permanently end my fertility at 34 years old, only two years into my marriage.

It's a surreal thing, isn't it?
Those of us who've received The Call know the sickening feeling.
Have you ever felt anything more disorienting?
The world gets really dark, really quickly.

On my diagnosis day, I was still awake at 3am. Exhausted, sore from my LEEP surgery *(Loop Electro-surgical Excision Procedure)* two days prior, my mind spinning, unable to sleep. So I began to write. From that day forward, I would often stay up late. I was afraid of the silence of night-time because the chatter in my mind would get so much louder. The pain in my soul was so deep I was certain heartache would kill me before my cancer could. But whenever I took out my laptop and wrote out my deepest feelings and made to-do and what-if lists to help myself make sense of things, the intensity of those dark moments drastically lessened and I would be able to finally fall asleep.

I hope that by sharing some of my writing from my journey with cervical cancer, you might feel seen, known, and have a friend who has been down this same road, accompanying you through your experience. I also hope that by sharing what I learned along the way, you can feel empowered and strong, with a plan to conquer cervical cancer and come out healthy in mind, body, and spirit.

I want this book to be a force of light in your own cancer darkness; something that pushes hope through when you can't find your way out of the shadows. These pages are yours to make your own. Draw pictures. Make lists. Write notes. I hope this little book becomes your constant companion.

andrea bonhiver
cervical cancer survivor

mantras

- I did not bring this upon myself. This is not my fault.
- Feelings aren't forever. Nor are they facts.
- Losing my female body parts does not make me less of a woman.
- I will not Google my symptoms. No matter what.
- I will seek support in whatever ways I can.
- I will do my best to be vulnerable with others.
- I will take care of myself before others. No excuses.
- I will ask for help and I will graciously receive it.
- I am not responsible for other people's emotions.
- I will honor my experience and be open to what I can learn.
- I will not 'should' myself. I will accept myself and my emotions.
- My pain is not too much for those around me.
- There is a well of strength and bravery in me. I can do this.
- I have cancer. Cancer does not have me.

introduction

Having met many cervical cancer patients and survivors online and a few in person, I know that it's common to feel curious about other patients' and survivors' stories leading up to their cervical cancer diagnosis. We look for shared experiences. I'll start by sharing my story with you.

After a routine pap smear in June 2017, HPV lesions (types 16 and 18) were found on my cervix. They were at the lowest level possible (CIN1), however my primary care physician recommended I have a colposcopy. This was a traumatic experience for me; one I'll never forget. The results still came back as CIN1, so my PCP recommended that we keep an eye on it and retest in a year.

In June 2018, I had another pap smear and those HPV lesions had advanced to CIN3. My PCP seemed concerned at the speed at which things had progressed, and another colposcopy was scheduled. The colposcopy results came back as only CIN1, which was confusing for me, initially. However, my PCP explained that all it meant was that she unfortunately didn't biopsy the area of my cervix where the CIN3 lesions were that the pap smear had picked up.

Since the pap had picked up CIN3, she recommended that we escalate the situation to a gynecologist and schedule a LEEP (Loop Electrosurgical Excision Procedure). Sometimes women are sedated for this procedure; I however was not. It was a painful and frightening experience that I still struggle to cope with today.

The biopsy that was taken during the LEEP revealed CIN3 as well as AIS (adenocarcinoma in situ) at the 12 o'clock spot on my cervix. The gynecologist called two days after the LEEP to slowly and gently share with me that this was considered Stage 0 cancer, and I would need a hysterectomy soon to prevent it from becoming more invasive.

After my diagnosis, I started searching for support groups online. I quickly learned that there are some women who have been diagnosed with cervical cancer at higher stages who do not consider AIS to be cancer. This was incredibly confusing to me. If it wasn't truly cancer, why did I need to see an oncologist? Why did I need an urgent hysterectomy?

So I did more research and talked with my oncologist. The American Cancer Society® classifies AIS as Stage 0 cancer and my oncologist treats it as such, as well. I never wanted to have to say, "I have cancer." So if it truly wasn't, I would've been glad about that. Unfortunately, it was cancer.

I think our culture expects to see women look sick when they have cancer. Cervical cancer treatments tend to either intensely affect your physical appearance, or leave you looking how you've always looked but completely wreak havoc on you internally. Some of us need chemotheraphy and radiation, some of us need hysterectomies, some of us are eligible for fertility-sparing treatments and surgeries— there is no typical treatment approach for cervical cancer and each type of treatment leaves some kind of damage in its wake.

Most of the damage cervical cancer did to me was internal, both physically and mentally. I suffered from anxiety, panic attacks, and depression, intense fatigue, difficulty remembering and focusing, and my cervix, uterus, and fallopian tubes were taken from me. I was sterilized. I bear two scars on my pelvis and the appearance of my belly button is permanently altered. I have nightmares. I struggle with exercise due to lingering issues with physical pain and mental trauma. I struggle with feeling feminine or womanly. My treatment wasn't poison in my veins; it was knives in my pelvis. There's really no point in comparison. None of us chose this and we are all grieving the unfair loss of many things.

It has taken some time for me to be comfortable calling myself a cancer survivor because I didn't need chemotherapy or radiation. I had a great deal of survivor's guilt when I was declared cancer free. Whenever anyone has called me strong, I've corrected them. I haven't felt strong because I was very negative and sad throughout my cancer journey, and I was always terrified of the next thing and the what ifs.

But this experience has taught me that we all survive cancer in a myriad of ways. Through our varied treatments of course, but also spiritually and mentally. Some of us are full of positivity and upbeat, even during the darkest seasons. Some of us fall apart and isolate. Regardless of how we get through it, the point is that we *do what it takes to get ourselves through it*. And we should never fault ourselves for it; we should celebrate ourselves for it. Because it is the definition of strength. There's so much strength in how we cope. There's strength in admitting something hurts and calling your doctor. There's strength in admitting you're not okay and scheduling a therapy appointment. There's strength in putting on that happy face because you know it's what's going to get you through the day.

I want to affirm you and your journey, regardless of your diagnosis, your prognosis, your stage, your coping mechanisms, or your treatment plan. We are in the thick of this together, feeling and experiencing many of the same things. I hope you feel welcomed into this sisterhood you never asked to be part of, and loved and supported deeply.

You can do this, dear sister.
You're stronger than you know.

telling people you have cancer

How do you break loved ones' hearts in an instant? Tell them you have cancer. It's the worst job. It can feel incredibly overwhelming to share the news of your diagnosis with family, friends, and coworkers. It's a complicated and nuanced activity that brings up a lot of layered emotions for all involved.

In the next few pages, I'll share a few of my journal entries from the early days of my diagnosis, where I was processing the experience of sharing my news with those around me, and the different ways in which people responded to it, as well as still processing the news myself. I hope it helps you make sense of some of your feelings around this unfair thing cancer forces all of us into.

Aug 4, 2018 // 2 am

It's 2:05am.
I just emailed 6 of my closest friends and told them that I have cancer.
I emailed them.
It's impersonal. Not exactly the best way to share news like this. I tried to be a little witty at first. Maybe a little funny and charming. To soften the impending blow.

How many times can you announce your cancer diagnosis and answer all of everyone's questions? I spent the last 24 hours doing just that. I'm so tired.

Everyone does a Caringbridge site. I mean, can you even really have cancer if you don't start a Caringbridge blog? It's just as impersonal as email. But in our fancy technological modern age—is it just as personal as a phone call? I'm quickly learning that informing and updating friends and family is a BIG job and it's not one I am entirely sure I want to manage.

Having cancer on social media is something I wish I didn't have to make a decision about.

It's just one of many decisions overwhelming me at the moment. I've known that I have cervical cancer for 24 hours now and I'm already unable to sleep, pouring over the mental checklist I need to attack in order to get to the place I want to be more than anywhere else—Living a life that isn't entirely consumed by the words that have run through my brain and stumbled off my lips constantly for the past day—adenocarcinoma in situ. On repeat.

I have to inform so many people. Family. Close friends. Some friends might be upset that I told other friends before them. "Why didn't you call me sooner?!" is something I've already heard. I've literally known for 24 hours. And I needed a little time to, I don't know…fall apart. Cry with my husband, Justin. Pull myself back together. And realize…I need to tell people, now. I have to figure out how to tell my boss that…

"I have cancer."
What a fun three words those are to drop into a room.

I've done it 6 times now in 24 hours and my heart doesn't race any less with each chance I get to practice.

I have to figure out how to take time off from work to recover from two upcoming surgeries. What's FMLA? Short-term disability? PTO? What's best? Can I trust HR? Will they hire a temp who will somehow phase me out of my position? Gotta worry about all of those things until I have an ulcer. Added to checklist.

I have to really confirm if the recommended oncologist I'll be seeing is actually in-network with our insurance. I called my health insurance company today in a ten minute gap I had between "I have cancer" meetings with family and friends, and the person on the phone couldn't entirely confirm if she's in-network or not. So I need to find time to figure that out. Or find another oncologist…

I have to read Google all the way to the last page to make sure I have learned everything there is to learn about adenocarcinoma in situ and how quickly it can progress and how long it will take me to heal from the cone biopsy that my gynecologist thinks my oncologist will want to do next, and what it will be like to recover from my hysterectomy.

Oh yes. I also need a hysterectomy. So. I need to get mentally and emotionally ready for that. 6-8 beautiful weeks on our bony old sectional sofa. Mostly with my dog as company. Which will be really nice most days because I enjoy quiet and puppy snuggles. But I know I will get lonely. And scared. And sad. Because I won't have a uterus anymore. And the nail has been permanently pounded in on my baby box. It'll be buried. Gone. Done. I'll still be a woman. But without most of the organs that many women feel makes them most female. Just tumbleweeds in there. And two stale ovaries housing what few eggs this almost-34-year old has left, JUST IN CASE I feel like having ANOTHER invasive surgery to harvest those eggs and try to get a surrogate pregnant. Awesome. Everything I ever dreamed of. Gotta decide if we're open to surrogacy or just really all-in on adoption. I feel good about adoption but I mean we should really weigh all of our options, right? Research, research, research! Added to checklist.

My college roommate sent a group text to the 8 of us that lived together way back when, this evening. It was a picture of her adorable 9-ish month old baby boy, asking us to come over and meet him. I love those girls and the friendship we had in college. Several girls replied, excited to get together. I wanted to. I wanted to say how ridiculously cute her son is and how I stalk her photos of him on Instagram all the time. Yeah, I want to come over and meet him and see her house and hang out with everyone and catch up. But. When we go around the room and talk about everything, I'll burst into tears. Because the baby and the house and the settled-in-ness symbolizes what I'm grieving right now. A uterus in place. A biological child. Young-family bliss. I'd so rather be back on the track to THAT place than on this detour to cancer station. It hurts a little. And I didn't want to drop any more bombs of sadness today. So I didn't reply. But I know I have to tomorrow. And the never-ending cancer to-do list continues to grip me awake tonight.

I want to call my grandmas. I want to hear Nanny's voice on the phone. And I want to squish into one of Grandma Diane's fleshy hugs. They're both gone now.

My longtime friend and his wife are expecting a baby. They announced it on Facebook the same day I found out about my cancer. I cried when I saw their announcement. Then I hated myself. I added, "Congratulate them," to my checklist. Gotta get to that one soon. Sometime. I really am happy for them. Thrilled. But the irony cut through me. And I just couldn't.

I want to undo all of this somehow. Rewind. Snap out of this dream. Burn my checklist. Give it to someone else to dispose of. The reality aches. And it's loud. I wish I could turn the volume all the way down, close my eyes, and drift to sleep.

August 5 // 8:54 pm

I spent the past 4 days trying to get used to saying the words, "I have cancer".
I have moments of almost inappropriate nonchalance. Other moments of heaviness and anxiety.
I've swung wildly between those extremes and rarely found myself in a peaceful in-between.
The uncontrollable explosion of tears and heaving sobs after I got the phone call was so unpleasant…I haven't been able to cry since.

I've slept. But not much. I wake up on the edge of a panic attack and have to talk myself down.
I don't even really know what I'm afraid of. I know that anxiety doesn't ALWAYS boil down to fear, but it often does. It isn't necessarily a fear of the usual things—being sick, throwing up, needles, blood, the unknown, passing out, pain… It's maybe loss of control?

It's probably partly due to also being forced into vulnerability. I like to be real and not keep secrets and feel like I can be honest about my life, no matter the setting or with whom. But this feels different.

I know that this news is mine to share and no one needs to know. But I do think that it's part of friendship to be honest and share things vulnerably.

So I have been revealing this news to close friends every few hours since Thursday night. Everyone has been so supportive. Although I've also found that I need to help some of them calm down. That frustrated me at first, but then I remembered that everyone takes news like this differently and they're entitled to their individual response. (Although, the more emotional someone gets the more fear I feel about what's ahead. Somehow the deeply-caring-yet-positive responses have helped me the most.)

I also realized that other people's anxieties are contagious; the people who react to this news with big emotions. I'm figuring out that I have to actually be mindful of what I take in from these interactions in order to maintain my mental and emotional health. No one else can do that for me. It's just hard to find the energy right now.

I have two more bomb-dropping sessions left. I have scheduled a meeting at 9am tomorrow with my boss. He knows I've been taking a few days away here and there this summer for what I've been simply referring to as, "outpatient medical procedures," but I haven't shared much beyond that. I'm pretty sure he thinks I've been going on job interviews.

I'll have to look at his face and say those three surreal words out loud again—I have cancer. In fact, this will be the first time I've told anyone to their face. With everyone else so far, it's been by phone, text, or email. I'm also going to tell my main coworker friend over our lunch hour. Every time I think of it my heart starts skipping beats in the heaviest way.

I don't know how they'll react, but I do know that I'll probably be really guarded and downplay it a bit and act very cool and collected about it. But I'm going to try REALLY HARD to dig down deep and be real. I want to appear strong and unphased and very capable most of the time. I don't know if it's an oldest-child trait or what. I like to keep things even-keeled. I don't like emotional outbursts. Having them or witnessing them. Maybe it's my German/Norwegian heritage. All of that put together makes sitting in a raw, vulnerable position with people I'm mainly in a professional relationship with, very nerve-wracking.

No matter how I act in those meetings, my instant reaction is going to be to come down hard on myself for being awkward or too guarded or too open. I should just decide right now that I'm entitled to act however I want to act and whatever comes naturally is just fine.

There's no right or wrong way to respond when people react to the news that I have cancer, and their emotions or judgments of me in that moment are not my responsibility to address or manage.

I'll also be getting a call tomorrow from the oncologist I've been referred to. We'll set up the first consultation and/or the cone biopsy. I'm nervous about that, since it's step one and it will feel really real all over again. The rawness of Thursday night, when I got the call, has been softened a bit over the past few days. Time has been a salve. But I am emotionally bracing myself for that phone call. I don't know what bombs they'll drop on the other end. The fact that I'll get the call sometime during the workday and I'll have to run to find an empty conference room to take the call and try to act normal afterward as I continue the workday is giving me anxiety as well.

I know, I know - I don't have to hold it together! I can be vulnerable! No one would expect someone who just got a cancer diagnosis and found out they are going to have their lady parts surgically removed and their fertility ripped away to hold it together all the time!

But we all know that this is not the world we live in in corporate America. We are delightful and pleasant and professional and rarely show our real selves. It's jarring in that setting. We talk about what we did on the weekend, only sharing the good things, leaving out the bad.

If I accidentally cried at work, I swear I'd run to the elevator and go directly to my car and drive straight home. I'd text my boss and tell him I wasn't feeling well and needed to leave. He'd be fine with that. But I'm sure the more that kind of thing occurs, the worse I'll look at work. I have to find a way to manage my work responsibilities, my fears, my emotions, my health, my treatment, and family and friends who want to help support Justin and I through this. It's so much.

It really still feels like a bad dream. SURREAL. I'm still saying, "I guess this is real," 10 times a day. I guess it has only been 4 days. But I bet 40 years post-hysterectomy, I'll probably still be saying it.

Justin has been just perfect. He is present. He is loving. He is caring. He has cooked two amazing dinners while I've been recovering from the LEEP, and two tasty breakfasts. He drove me to a coffee shop and vintage store so I could check out a sale, and just waited in the car. He's helping me keep things light and made a funny joke about everyone wanting to give me gifts and take me out to lunch and dinner and coffee. It's, "Congratulations! You have cancer!" or "Happy Cancer!" as he sarcastically remarked when he brought me breakfast in bed on Friday morning. He knew I had a day ahead of me where I'd be rehashing the cancer diagnosis and all of the science and the prognosis and my feelings and emotions to my two close friends who obviously just want to be supportive and ask more questions. But it can be draining. Can I feel drained and depleted but grateful and loving at the same time? It's how I feel.

I always want to remember having coffee with Allie and Lindsay that day. The sweet card from Allie and the heartfelt words. Lindsay gave me permission to be real and honest and be sad and mad if I need to. Because I was so dried up from all the talking and emotion of the previous days, I sounded VERY matter-of-fact about having cancer and I think she thought I was holding back. But I so appreciated her verbalizing that it was a safe space to be whatever I needed to be. I could talk to those two about what I'd be losing by not carrying a child and be sad about that with them but also be really honest about every feeling I have regarding that topic. I love that I can have the realest conversations with those two. And they go on for hours and even though it exhausts this introvert, they are always so meaningful and special and I am so grateful for them.

My brother Chad took Justin and I out for dinner. We did a lot of reminiscing and laughing, which is what my family always does. Even though he's currently unemployed, he bought us dinner, plus drinks and dessert. He wanted to do something. And I can tell he is affected and wanting to help. He texted me several times after dinner wanting to help with HR stuff and helping me understand how to take a leave from work. I am grateful for my little brother. My longest relationship. My oldest friend. We look out for each other.

I feel so overwhelmed. I'm sure Justin does too. In totally different ways than I do. Seeing me in such a rough state, not really knowing how to support me, etc. He probably also has his own anxieties about my health. And our future. I don't know how to support him or what to watch for to be sure he's ok and handling everything well. What can I do for him? I really don't want to just take, take, take from him and not be able to give anything but a thank you in return...it's not enough.

My heart and mind and mouth are exhausted from all the talking. The crying. The NOT SLEEPING. But I lie awake playing out scenarios, rehearsing how I'll interact with coworkers once they hear the news...will they treat me differently? Will everyone come over and say SORRY and I'll have to like, look at their faces and welling-up eyes and not know how to respond besides, "Thanks"? Ugh.

But I know I need to sleep for my health. It's just so difficult to shut off my mind. It's honestly never been more difficult. With all the struggles I've had in my life with falling asleep at night, the only other time I can ever remember this pain in my heart and my racing thoughts keeping me awake, is right before and right after my dear friend Christie died of brain cancer five years ago. That physical pain of grief. And the playground that gets built in your mind. The minute you hit the pillow, you just jump on that creaky old merry-go-round and hold on tight while the wind blows you in a circle. You're so dizzy as you look around, but every once in awhile, the blurry landscape around you stops and your eyes grab hold of something: a new topic. Topic after topic after topic after topic. You can't get off that ride. As much as you REALLY want to.

Well...T-11 hours until I'll be at work, sitting in my boss' office, dropping my bomb again. I woke up panicking every 2-3 hours last night. I really hope I can get some rest. Sleeping pills just make it harder to wake up in the morning, so I really don't want to take one. I need your magic sleeping pills, God. Please help me. Peace in my chest...and rest.

time to process

What has been the hardest part about telling those around you that you have cancer?

Are you holding yourself responsible for others' emotions? If so, write about letting that go, below. Free yourself from that weight.

What has been the most helpful or supportive response that you've received from someone in your life?

telling people you have cancer

Use these next several open pages to reflect and process your experience of telling others that you have cancer, all while absorbing the news of your diagnosis in your own heart and mind. Write about the responses that helped you. It might also help to write about what kind of reactions hurt or weren't helpful. Write about how it made you feel to tell your loved ones that you have cancer.

telling people you have cancer

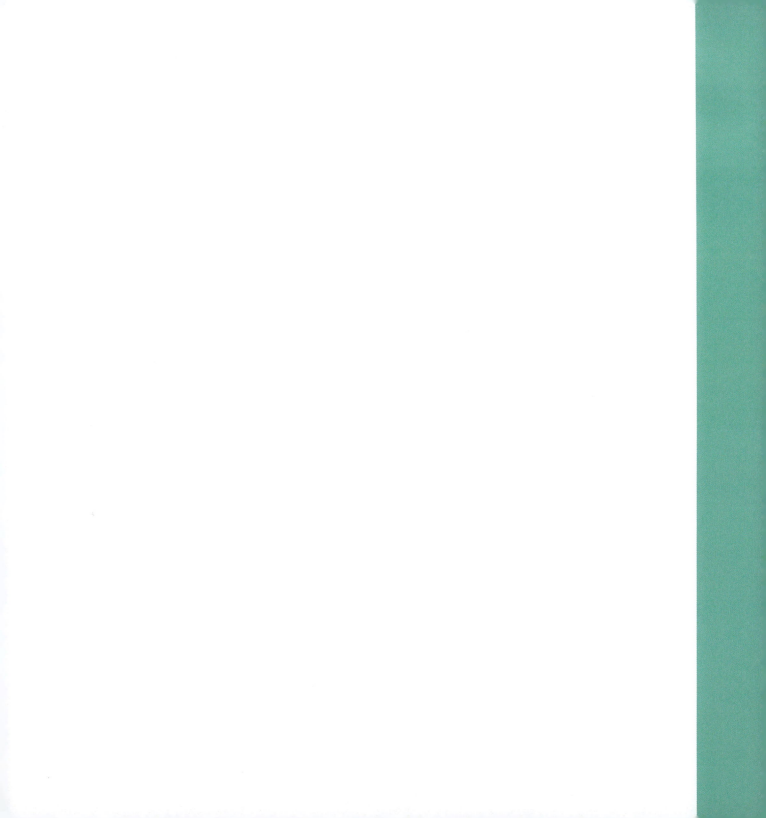

telling people
you have cancer

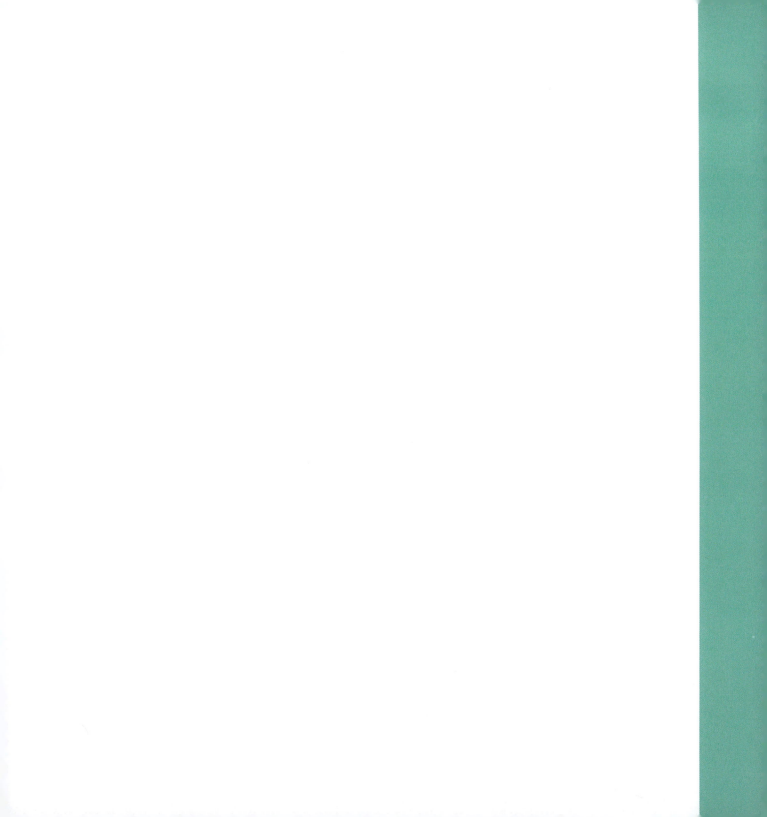

telling people you have cancer

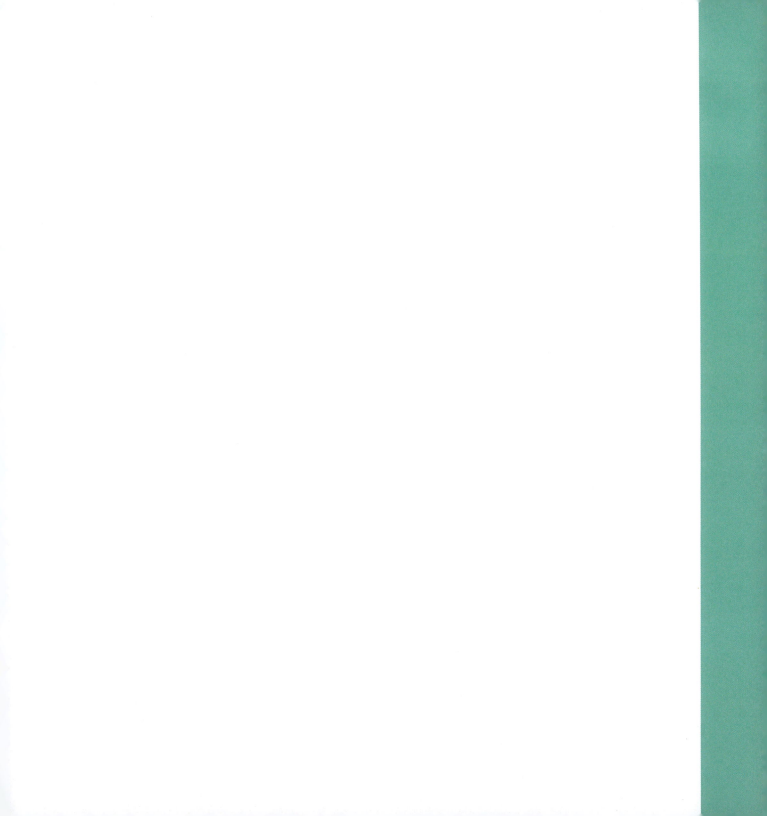

telling people you have cancer

telling people you have cancer

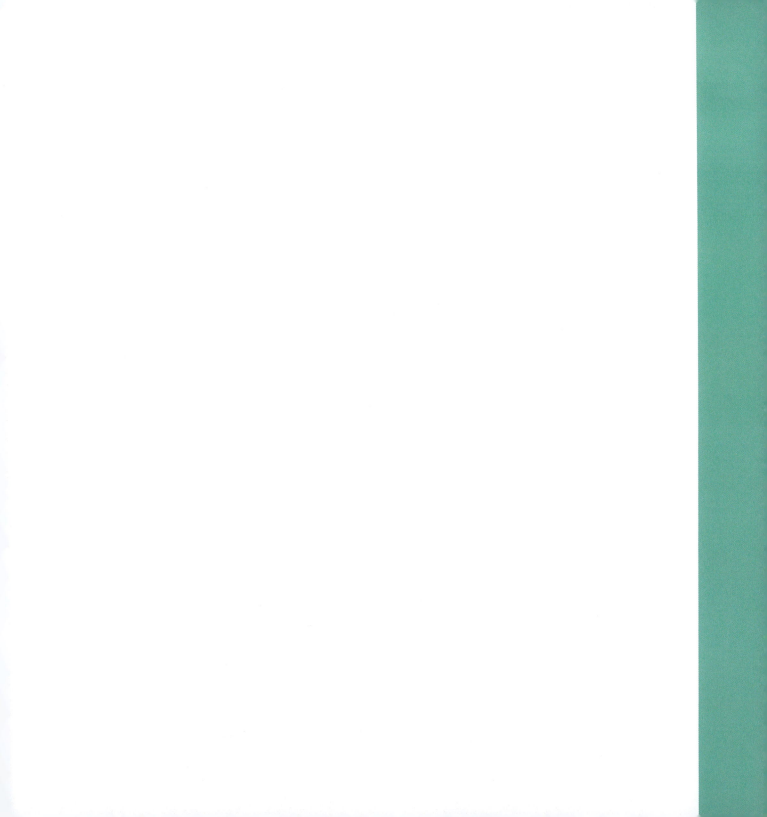

telling people you have cancer

your first oncology appointment

If there's any gap of time between your diagnosis and your first oncology appointment, it can be excruciating. There's a lot of unknowns to face and the idea of waiting for vital information and questions to be answered is anxiety-inducing and exhausting.

The fact that you need to see an oncologist is likely very jarring and overwhelming. In the next few pages, I'll share some of my journaling about my first oncology appointment. I hope that by sharing my experience, it will take some of the fear of the unknown and mystery away from what you're in for at your first visit, as well as help you discover some good coping strategies for the fear and anxiety that inevitably comes with setting foot in a cancer center.*

*My experience is a good general point of comparison for this experience. However, everyone's diagnosis is different and comes with a different care plan and recommended approach. My oncologist's perspective will likely not be the same as yours, nor will my exact experience be reflective of your own. Each of us will have varied experiences based on our unique situation.

August 20 // 1:45pm

The oncology appointment was last Tuesday. My anxiety level heading into it was off the charts. I took a little anti-anxiety medication the night before and again the morning of, took 1ml CBD oil before leaving for the appointment, a little more anti-anxiety medication in the waiting room, dabbed lavender oil on my wrists and under my nose, and prayed like heck that I'd make it through.

My mom came with me and we met my mother-in-law Susan there. Susan offered to come along and take notes. She's a recently retired oncology nurse so I absolutely welcomed her! I knew my brain was going to shut down soon after we got there.

Right when we got off the elevator, a woman was standing there with no hair. No eyebrows, lashes, peachfuzz on her face...nothing. She looked so tired. I met eyes with her and we smiled small smiles at each other.

I sat down in the waiting room and filled out more paperwork while my mom and Susan quietly caught up with one another.

They called my name and I went back to the exam room alone. The nurse that took my vitals was pretty crappy at her job. I guess I'm used to kind nurses. She did not care about me at all. She was blatantly annoyed with me, making eye-rolling faces if I didn't answer her questions exactly the way she wanted me to, only looking at the computer screen and not once at my face. She left me in the room alone and told me to get completely undressed quickly. I put on the gown and sat on the bed staring at the floor in a daze. Where the hell was I? Why did I have to be there?

Another nurse came in. This one didn't have scrubs on. She wore normal clothes. She is kind of an administrative nurse for my oncologist. Her name is Anne. She went through more of my medical history with me and verified things from my paperwork. She was much kinder to me. Much softer and more understanding and empathetic. After that, she said she'd be back in with the oncologist soon.

My doctor's name is Emily. We're about the same age, which is kind of crazy to think about. But I liked her a lot. She was positive and upbeat but also didn't sugarcoat anything. She did a quick pelvic exam with Anne holding the light for her, and mentioned that a blood vessel was nicked during the LEEP, which explained the scary bleeding I had in the days leading up to that appointment. She said it looked like it was closing back off on its own and everything was healing well so I had nothing to worry about. It was really nice to get that reassurance. I didn't need a blood draw, either, which I was relieved about.

She then invited my mom and Susan back to the room. She laid out the situation like this: AIS *(Adenocarcinoma in situ)* was found on my cervix at the 12 o'clock spot. The LEEP removed it and the margins were pretty clear. Because of that, she was comfortable with not doing a cone biopsy right now. (What a relief).

However, she drew a diagram and explained how AIS has something called skip cells that can show up deeper and in other random spots in the pelvis in unpredictable patterns, causing cancer in other parts of the body. It doesn't metastasize like other types of cancer, which is why I need a hysterectomy to stop it in its tracks, and she advised me to not wait longer than a year to have the surgery.

But since I'm young, she really wanted me to think long and hard about doing the hysterectomy right away, or trying to have a baby first. It would mean starting to try NOW, and getting more-than-regularly-scheduled paps and colposcopies, just to make sure AIS isn't suddenly becoming more invasive. I'd have to be monitored really closely. Then 6 weeks after the birth, I'd have the hysterectomy. She then laid out the other approach for just getting the hysterectomy right away and talking about surrogacy or adoption.

My mom and Susan each asked my doctor their questions. Susan took notes. Then when the oncologist left the room at the end, my mom asked,

"So what are you initially thinking you want to do?" I was flooded with information. I don't want to do ANY. OF. THIS.

I assumed my mom either was hoping I'd tell her I want to have her grandkids first, or that I want this cancer removed ASAP. Two answers I was nowhere near prepared to give. Especially candidly in front of both of them.

Susan left and my mom and I met Dad for lunch to fill him in. He seemed stressed out. I understand this is all happening to my parents too. But man. It sucks for me to have to watch this wreak emotional havoc on them and not feel somehow responsible.

At lunch, I had an Old Fashioned and some pizza. Comfort. The cocktail got me talking a bit and I said a lot about adoption. My parents were being supportive of whatever I was thinking and trying to be positive for me. But I think in my heart of hearts that they really would rather have an adopted grandkid (or no grandkid) than lose me. It seems like their desired plan is for me to have the hysterectomy right away. At lunch, that was pretty much my thought too. The fear in this situation is so very acute and strong and it bubbles up with such intensity, that it makes me want to just end this mess as soon as possible and have everything taken out right away.

That night, I filled Justin in on the details from my appointment and we decided to just not talk about it any more that night and relax. The next morning, I couldn't get out of bed. 9am rolled around and I hadn't even contacted work. I decided to shoot my boss an email and let him know that the appointment went well but I had some phone calls to make and wanted privacy, so I'd be working from home.

I spent the day doing a little bit of work, but mostly watching YouTube videos about surrogacy, adoption, researching costs, talking to my oncologist's office and asking if eggs could be harvested during a hysterectomy or if it had to be a separate operation, calling fertility clinics, my health insurance company for estimates, and just generally losing my damn mind. I made chaotic, scrambled lists in a notebook like someone having a psychotic break.

That night, Justin and I went to a luau party at our favorite local restaurant patio, Longfellow Grill.

I had two Mai Tais. I had never had one before. Turns out one will flatten you. Two will make you sob your face off on the couch because you have cancer and it's not fair and this decision is impossible to make.

Justin and I had a LONG talk that night. Well, he talked. I cried mostly. I talked some. We got really honest. We vetoed surrogacy and decided that maybe... God has given us this little final window of time. We realized that down the line, we would both probably regret it if we never even gave it a shot. Cancer is a real fear. It's valid. But with close monitoring, MAYBE it won't get worse while we try for a baby. Since that fear is looming, we agreed on a time frame to try for. So we'll try to get pregnant for 6-7 months, then regroup with my oncologist and see if we could keep trying if we're not pregnant yet, or if the hysterectomy is needed right away.

So because this decision is highly personal and I don't want to be forced into sharing so widely that we're going to try for a baby, I deleted the Caringbridge page I had started but hadn't yet posted anywhere. I have told a few girl friends that we're going to try for a baby for awhile (since they know about the cancer and want to be updated), but we kept things very vague with our parents. We just wanted to control some portion of this, so we didn't tell them what we're doing, but said we've given ourselves a timeframe to decide on when to do the hysterectomy and we will share it with them once we've arrived at a decision. They can draw their own conclusions about what's going on over these next 6 months.

I know it takes a lot of couples a long time to get pregnant. Especially after being on birth control pills for many years. But I'm trusting that my oncologist will take good care of me, and I'm stepping into something scary and unknown and seeing what God will do in this time. If it's not a baby that comes out of it, it will be something else to learn and appreciate. I'm putting my faith in that.

And yes. I'm terrified of being pregnant. Always have been. But I guess maybe I became more terrified of living the rest of my life, knowing we maybe had a chance to have a biological kid and didn't take it. I'd always wonder what our unique brand of kid would be like. And Justin said he'd always wonder about it too. So we have to step into this and put fear aside, focusing on the goodness of God and the fact that we are supported by many friends and family.

So we're giving it our all. I have an app tracking my fertile days. I'm taking the most disgusting but most highly rated prenatal vitamins I could find. I'm trying to drink more water. I'm only having one glass of red wine a week (those Mai Tais turned out to be my final cocktails for awhile!). I'm trying to relax and stress less (easier said than done when one has cancer slowly growing in their body). I'm starting to exercise again now that the LEEP healing is mostly done. My point in all this being: we are going to give it our BEST SHOT. So that when 6 months is up, we know that we really tried our best and don't have to look back at this time like we threw away our only chance.

According to my oncologist, if I'm pregnant and the cancer starts to become more invasive, I may end up on bedrest in the hospital, possibly having a cone biopsy and monitored even more closely. Every pregnancy comes with risks, so I'm choosing to look at that as a normal possibility, not an additional risk. Any pregnant woman could end up on hospital bedrest.

And if it doesn't work out for us—we both feel comfortable with adoption. Or a different plan for our future, and maybe we'll figure that out later.

It's been a LOT to process. But I'm feeling lighter since we made the decision. Less angry. Less afraid. More supported and strong. I had gotten approval from my doctor to increase my antidepressant. I started to titrate up for one day, then decided not to. Maybe I feel so much lighter right now because even though we didn't really choose any of this mess, we seized this chance to take control of this one thing. ONE thing.

time to process

How did you feel before and after your first visit to the oncologist? How did you cope?

Were you presented with any big decisions to be made at your appointment? What were they and what was that like?

What would you like to have more control over? What are you angry about?

your first oncology appointment

Use these open pages to reflect and process your experience of going to the oncologist for the first time, and any additional medical appointments you've had so far. Consider writing about some of the decisions you may have to make regarding your treatment and the future of your body.

your first oncology appointment

what if

Fear and worry were the themes of my existence when I had cancer. I mean, how can they not be? There's so much control that gets ripped away when you're diagnosed. You have no idea how this story will end. You might feel alone. You're likely grieving the loss of many things, physical and intangible.

Soon after my diagnosis, I started seeing my therapist on a weekly basis. I had been going off and on throughout my 20s, but knew it would be important to see her more often during this cancer journey to help me with my anxiety. Anxiety and depression often go together, one feeding into the other. At one visit, she challenged me to really take an honest look at what she called my "black undercurrent" and start naming the things that pulled me under. The purpose of the exercise was to learn to identify the darkest places of my mind and how to not let those places push me into depression.

I'll share some of those places with you, here. Maybe you can relate in your own way, in your unique situation.

- I see myself on a hospital bed. No makeup. Feeling very anxious. Nauseated. Sweaty. Crying a little. IV in my arm. Wearing a hospital gown. Getting ready to be put under for surgery. Justin is to my right by my head. I'm thinking about how I always pictured him there as I gave birth. But he's just there to help me feel calm now as our chances of ever giving birth are ripped away. Just that image is enough to make me depressed.

- I see myself in a hospital bed. Waking up after surgery. Nauseous. Crying. But this time, not crying from fear. Crying from grief. Because my uterus will be gone. My fallopian tubes will be gone. My lymph nodes may be gone. And I will officially be unable to have a baby. Sterilized. The nails will be in the coffin. My entire life, I acted like I had a choice about having a baby or not. I acted like one day, I'd just do it and that would be that. I have a uterus and it's part of having a uterus. It gives you a baby. Having someone take it away is out of my control. It's not my choice. It's not what I want. It's very hard to come to terms with it.

- I see myself sitting on the couch at home. Justin is bringing me fizzy waters on ice. I feel ugly. Pale. Can't wear the false lashes that I'm so attached to wearing every day. I feel restless. Bored. Emotional. Angry and sad. Wishing I felt differently, for Justin and for myself. For the room. For our dynamic.

- I see myself sitting on the couch at home. My mom hands me a baby. It hurts to hold it. My core muscles are weak and sore. I grieve the fact that my mom has to be there to help so much and I can't even pick up my own baby and I wish Justin and I could have these special first weeks with our baby to ourselves. It's not what I wanted. And I feel more like a spectator than a participant. Stuck on the couch. In pain.

- What if we don't have a baby? In February, I get checked again and we schedule the hysterectomy.

- I have the hysterectomy. While I'm recovering, I get a call from the oncologist. They found higher stages of cancer. I need chemo/radiation. I am so terrified of it. Of the nausea, all the appointments, the blood work, the fatigue, the long-term issues. I don't want to be sick.

- I have the hysterectomy. We don't have a baby. I don't have a uterus. And when they biopsy my organs, they don't find any more cancer. Cancer free, baby-free, uterus free. What DO I have then? No consolation prize? All the things get taken away? For what? Being cancer free is excellent. But the cost was massive.

- What if we can't have a baby and Justin feels let down. He'll never say it to me. But what if he harbors resentful thoughts for years? Maybe if I'd taken better care of myself or just relaxed or been less anxious we could've gotten pregnant.

- What if we can't have a baby and Justin blames himself. And I have to try to cheer him up when I'm so sad, too, and blaming myself. We'd both tell each other it's neither of our faults, but we'd tell ourselves it was all our fault. It would be a really negative, dark place to be.

- I'm afraid I'll get checked in February and they'll find more cancer or skip cells when they do the ECC *(Endocervical Curettage)*, and then I'll regret that we took this time to try for a baby. Is it insane to even assume we MIGHT be able to get pregnant in 6 months? I feel like that's really wishful thinking. It's rarely that easy for anyone. Part of me wishes I would've asked for the ECC back in August so I could know one way or another if I have any cancer cells in the cervical canal. If I ask for the ECC now, I'll have to wait 3 weeks to recover + a period somewhere in there, and that means we'd lose 1 or 2 chances to conceive. And we only have 4 left. So really, it's just too late for the ECC. I regret not asking for one in August. I wish the clock wasn't literally ticking on our chances at having a biological family.

- I'm scared of becoming bitter about this. I'm scared I'll play the victim for the rest of my life. I'm scared I'll get really overweight or have a spending problem or a drinking problem because I'll always use the excuse of, "I've been through a lot, I should go easy on myself. I deserve to get the things I want when I can."

- I'm afraid I'll wall myself off from friendships or from doing things I once enjoyed, like planning parties and entertaining. Because I'm too exhausted from all the negative things, there's nothing left to put into the positive.

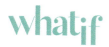

Use the following open pages to list your worst fears. Lay them all out. Don't hold back. Keep adding to the list as new ones arise. If you're feeling brave, vulnerably share these fears and worries with someone close to you. Ask them to help you come up with an, "If this happens, then…" solution for each one. Inviting someone into your world and creating a plan takes a lot of the power away from anxious thought patterns.

whatif

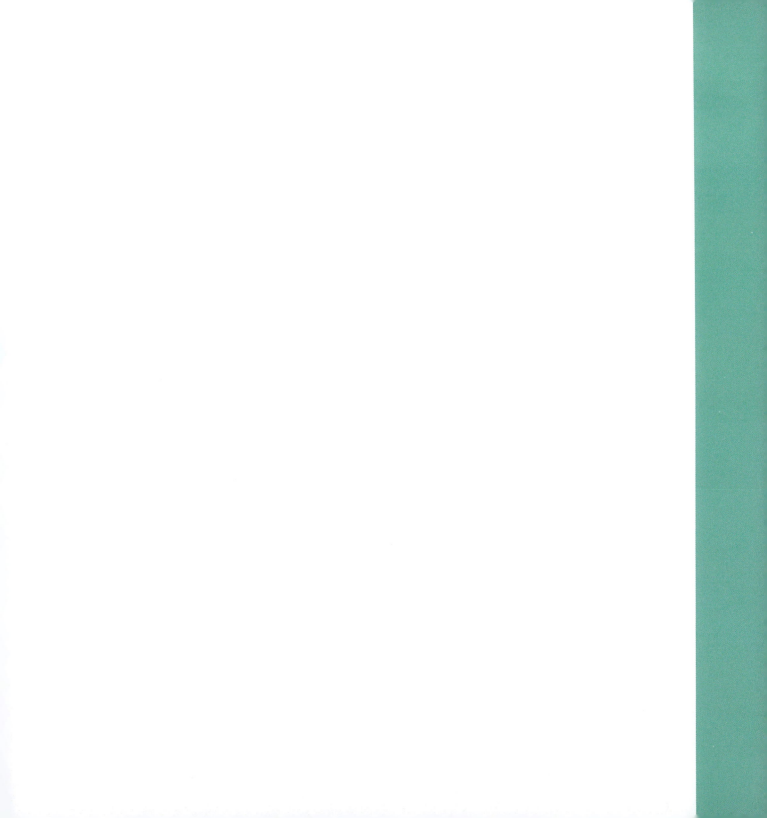

whatif

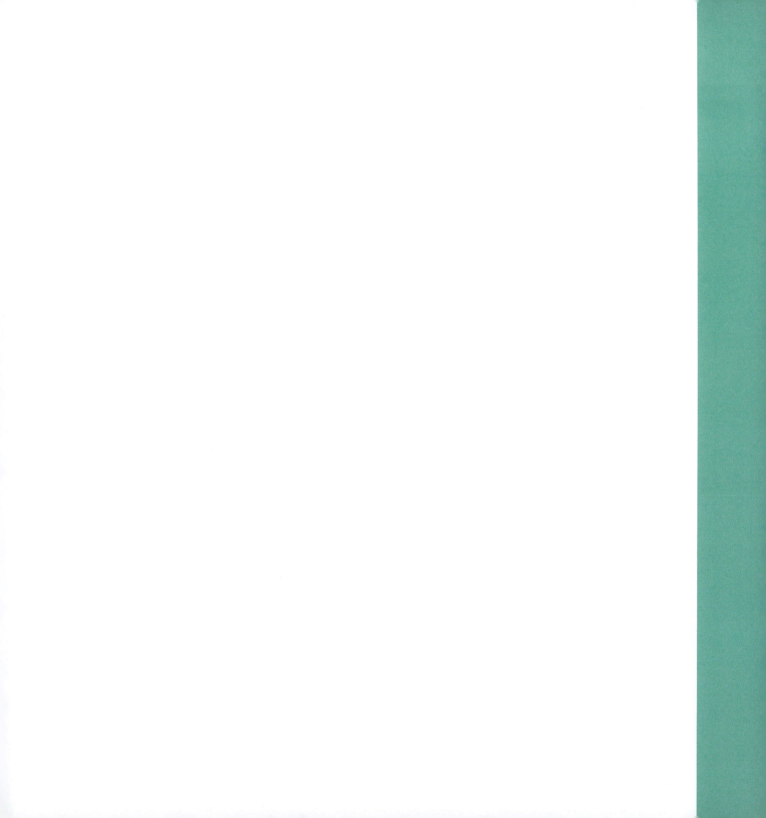

whatif

whatif

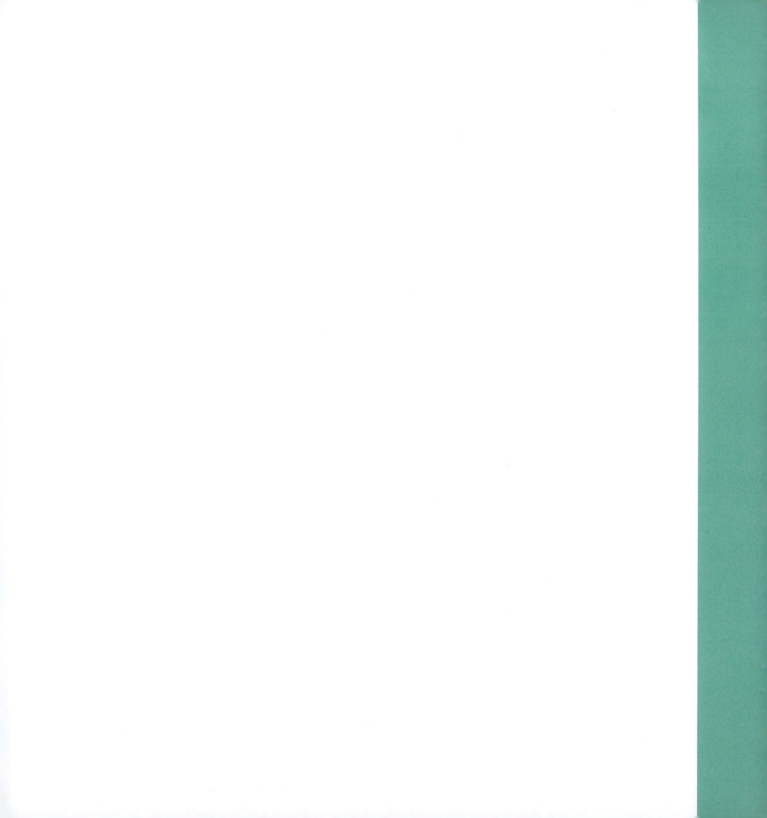

whatif

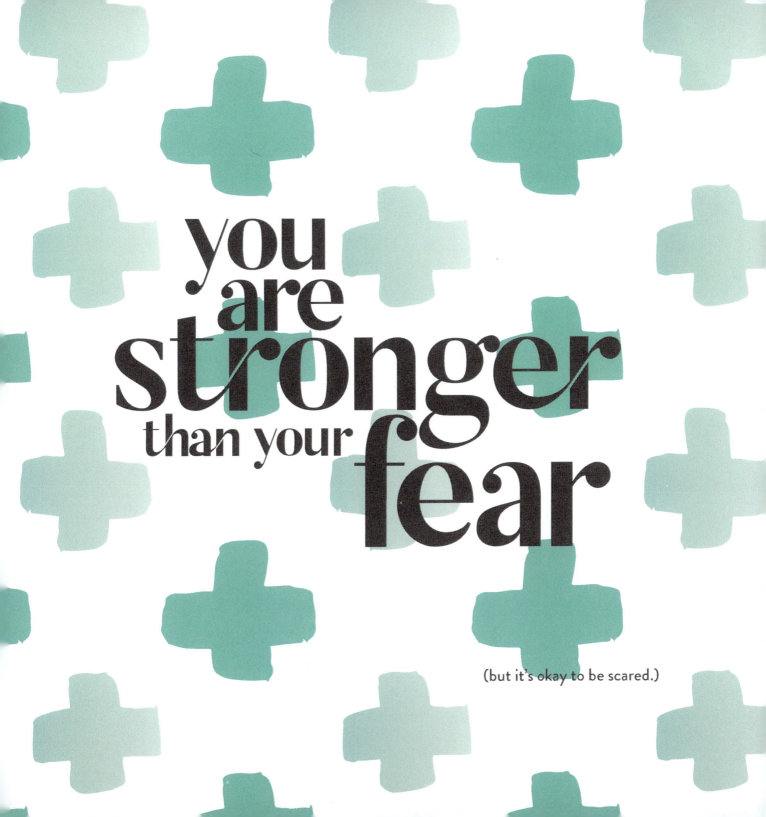

the facts

The trauma of being diagnosed with cancer can take a toll on cognition, and sometimes our memories don't work as well as we'd like. Especially if we begin chemotherapy or radiation or are recovering from surgery, we'll need help keeping track of important information.

During those dark nights when you're up late and your mind is spinning, refer back to these notes to remind yourself of what's true. There were a few nights right before my hysterectomy where I actually got out the paperwork from my last oncology visit just to fact-check that I hadn't misunderstood something along the way and that I actually *did* have cancer and *did* need the surgery.

Our minds can play tricks on us when we're overwhelmed and it's easy to make up stories when we're focused on fear. But we can ground ourselves by looking at the facts and trusting what we know to be true.

the facts

Use these open pages to take notes at each medical appointment. It can be helpful to ask a friend or family member to attend appointments with you and have them take notes for you. *Tip: Include the date and time with each note*

the facts

the facts

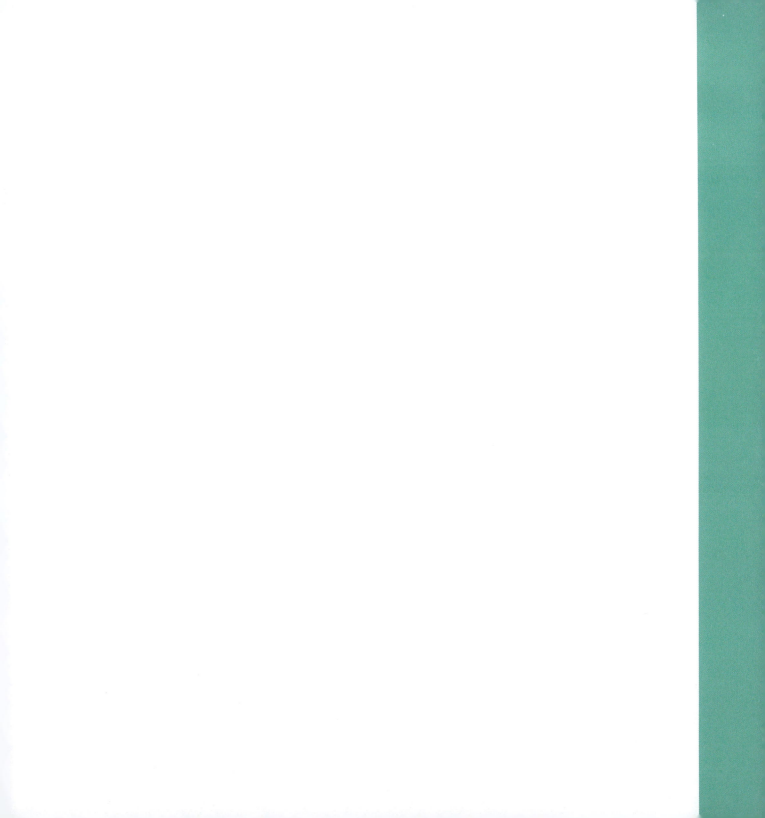

the facts

hpv facts

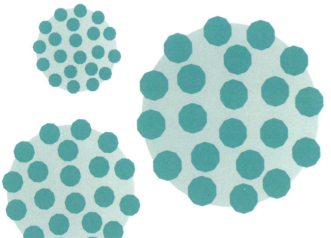

The human papilloma virus (HPV) can cause 6 types of cancer, including cervical cancer.

HPV is extremely common. More than 33,000 men and women get HPV in the United States each year. Four out of five people can expect to have it at one time or another. There are typically few if any symptoms.

HPV is not contracted only by people who have multiple sexual partners. It is not a sign of being promiscuous. HPV can be contracted after intimate contact with only one person.

There are no HPV tests for men, although they do carry and transmit it. Women are now tested for HPV at most annual pap smear exams. HPV types 16 and 18 are the types that most often cause cervical cancer. There is no way of knowing whose bodies will have immune systems that are able to clear the HPV virus independently, and whose HPV will mutate their cells into cancer. The only way to protect the population is by vaccination.

The HPV vaccine is well-tested, safe, and successful at preventing 90% of HPV infections that could lead to 6 types of cancer, including cervical cancer. The most common reactions from the vaccine are mild and like those of other vaccines.

The 2019 CDC guidelines for vaccination are as follows: Children and adults aged 9 through 26 years. HPV vaccination is routinely recommended at age 11 or 12 years; vaccination can be given starting at age 9 years. Catch-up HPV vaccination is recommended for all persons through age 26 years who are not adequately vaccinated. People through age 46 may also be vaccinated to help the body's immune response to HPV as they age.

cervical cancer facts

Women with early cervical cancers and pre-cancers usually have no symptoms. Symptoms often do not begin until the cancer becomes invasive and grows into nearby tissue.

When this happens, the most common symptoms are: Pain during sex, abnormal vaginal bleeding, such as bleeding after vaginal sex, bleeding after menopause, bleeding and spotting between periods, and having periods that are longer or heavier than usual. Bleeding after douching or after a pelvic exam may also occur.

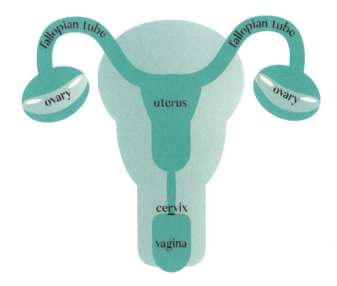

Cervical cancer is typically discovered via a protocol of testing involving an annual pap exam, a positive HPV result, a cervical biopsy, a more in-depth cervical sample (called a LEEP or cone biopsy), then a cancer diagnosis. Cervical cancer is treated by chemotherapy, radiation, and surgery.

According to the American Cancer Society®, of the 13,170 new cervical cancer diagnoses in the United States in 2019, about 4,250 women will die. The HPV vaccine prevents cervical cancer. The great hope is that with more people being vaccinated each year, there will soon come a day when we stop seeing this all-too-common preventable cancer altogether.

Tip: *Show friends and family members these pages when you're tired of explaining the details behind your diagnosis. It can be draining to have to educate those around you, so let me do the work for you! Consider sharing photos of these pages on social media to spread this knowledge and answer questions friends may be asking.*

mantras

- I will not expect myself to remember everything in great detail.

- I will call my oncologist without hesitation to ask questions and get clarification when I question the facts or can't recall details.

- I will take notes at every appointment or enlist a friend or family member to do it for me.

- I will decrease the number of things in my personal life that I need to remember to do, keep track of, organize, etc. I will create space for peace in my mind.

- I do not need to become an expert on cervical cancer. Google is available for everyone in the world, and if people have questions, they can do their own research. It is not my job to teach all the time.

- I will study the facts and trust them.

you will grow through this

(even if you're overwhelmed today.)

before treatment

When you already have cancer on your mind, adding surgery, recovery, chemo, radiation, and a list of to-dos and decisions to make is just about enough to push the average woman right over the edge. *You don't need that stress!*

When I had cancer, I was humbled by the number of people in my life who offered to step up and help in whatever ways that my husband and I needed. Many would say well-meant things like, "I'll do whatever you want. You just let me know!" Well, what I wanted was to *not have cancer* and to *not have to make any of these decisions*. I was suddenly the party planner for my own really weird and sad cancer event and I had to organize the guest list and give everyone jobs to do. I never interviewed for this role, I wasn't sure how I got hired, and I wanted to quit.

Whether it's a chemo and/or radiation, brachytherapy, a LEEP, a cone biopsy, a colposcopy, a trachelectomy, a radical hysterectomy or a total hysterectomy— It's easy to freak out. Many of us have to contend with a fear of medical procedures (If that's you, write or draw about it in the **What If** section of this journal), while many of us are also immediately faced with an onslaught of mental to-dos when we think about treatment and recovery. Who will take care of my children? Who will do the grocery shopping? Who will take over my projects at work? Will I lose my job? Am I eligible for paid leave? Will insurance cover this?

Wading through the to-dos and questions that need answers all alone is a terrible idea. But delegating is not easy and it can take its own toll. I hope the guided prompts in this section help you think through some topics that will get you to a place of peace and confidence before treatment begins.

February 18 // 12:19pm

I had a really hard time getting out of bed today. I kept thinking, "I don't want to do this day because it's taking me one day closer to the hysterectomy." It's like I want to freeze time. It feels like each day closer is sadder and sadder and scarier and scarier. I've gained a lot of tools to cope, but it still feels just giant. I wish I could stay in bed all day and put it off forever.

There's so much to do and think about and plan for. It's all overwhelming. I have this note open in my phone with all kinds of questions and checklists and things I need to do/clean/buy before surgery. I created and organized my own help calendar and shared it with Justin and our moms and Allie. Anytime anyone asks me a question about surgery and what I want, I want to freak out and yell at them. A) I'm overwhelmed and don't know the answer to your question. If I knew the answer to your question once, I forgot. Don't expect me to remember *anything*. B) I don't WANT any of this. Making choices is stressful, even about things that should make me feel better or give me something to look forward to after this is all over. (What kind of snacks or fizzy waters I want during recovery, etc.) If it meant I didn't have to have a hysterectomy, I'd never drink fizzy water again. These are things I don't care about and they aren't making me super extra happy. It's just another decision I have to make about something I don't want to do.

I'm feeling a little bit again like I did when this all started. How everyone comes at you with questions and things you have to respond to. Sometimes you have to spend time digging around or researching for information before you answer everyone. It's overwhelming. All the logistics and planning and communications. I don't like that kind of thing. I am so stressed out.

time to process

What are you most stressed out about currently?

Is there anyone in your life that you can delegate some of the overwhelming tasks to?

Is there any activity or commitment in your life that you can cut out during this time to alleviate your stress?

before treatment

Use this space to write out what's overwhelming you and begin to make a plan to tackle each item. Ask for help and accept it! Delegate whatever you can to your spouse or partner, family members, or a close friend.

practical prep

These are some helpful and practical things to do that can make you feel more in control of what's happening to you before treatment begins. Do not try to do these all in one day, although you may be tempted. Take your time, and if possible, delegate some of them to someone close to you.

- If you have insurance, call the number on the back of your card or visit the company website. Ask any questions you might have about coverage for your treatment, procedure, or surgery. If possible, pre-schedule a time with a representative so you don't feel rushed. There are also many health insurance companies with physical locations that you can visit.

- Discuss fertility preservation options with your doctor or ask for a fertility specialist referral, if you'd like to add to your family in the future. Depending on your diagnosis, sometimes alternatives to hysterectomies are an option, as well as preserving eggs. Speak with your oncologist about your options before contacting a fertility specialist.

- If you're having surgery, discuss post-op preferences with your doctor. Tell them about other surgeries you've had and how you tolerated the medications and anesthesia. Advocate for yourself and mention the things you're worried about. For me, it was feeling nauseous after surgery. My doctor assured me that she'd make notes for the nursing staff to give me extra anti-nausea medication and to send me home with more in case it became a problem. Knowing I could count on that took away a lot of my anxiety.

- If you are currently employed, set up a time to speak with your manager or the HR department about your eligibility for taking leave from work for treatment and/or surgery recovery. If possible, bring documentation from your oncologist and ask them to explicitly recommend a number of weeks that they want you to rest and recover.

- If you aren't currently connected with a support group for cervical cancer patients and survivors, this is the perfect time to join one. I highly recommend Cervivor™. They are an incredibly well-informed advocacy organization with a private, welcoming, and highly supportive social media group that you can participate in before, during, and after your cervical cancer journey. Members will share their experiences, give advice, and encourage you. Find them at cervivor.org and on social media.

ask for (and accept) help

You're used to doing it all.
This is often the hardest part of navigating through a medical interruption in a person's life. Accepting help from others is humbling, sometimes awkward, and can make us feel like a burden on those around us.

Let me assure you: *You are not a burden.* One of the most beautiful lessons you'll learn through this is that humans want to help other humans because they have been helped by other humans. Accept that help. And do not hesitate to ask for it. You don't know who in your life would be honored to be asked to lend a hand.

Who can you look to for support? Make a list below.
Consider those in your life who are closest to you or friends and family who may have already offered to help.

ways to ask

- Ask someone close to you if they would consider starting a Meal Train for you. Be honest with them if you feel uncomfortable asking, but voice that it would be very helpful and you think you might need the assistance.
- Contact your house of worship if you have one and tell them about your situation. They're likely very used to members asking for help and are usually more than willing to organize assistance.
- Call, text, or email close family members and ask if you can count on their help during treatment or surgery. Start an online calendar and give everyone access. Let them fill in their own availability.
- If you're active and open on social media, that may also be a good place to ask for help.

Tip: *When asking in writing, keep things short. Don't feel like you have to write a sob story or prove your worthiness. You have cancer! You deserve to be cared for. Be honest if you feel awkward putting yourself out there in this way, and be gracious toward anyone willing to offer you help.*

life goes on

It's a well-known fact that women make the world go 'round. We handle it. *All of it.*
Think about all of the things that you do to keep your life and household going and list them below. After you've listed all of the tasks, go back through and write down important things to know about each task so that whoever takes over this responsibility while you're recovering from surgery or on treatment days can refer to your notes. Follow the example below.

TASK: Feeding the dog
THINGS TO KNOW: Louis eats at 6am and 5pm. He gets 1/2 cup of the wet food stored on the top pantry shelf. He is fine to wait for his meal an hour or so later than those times. Louis should not be given treats or human food. His favorite toy is the stuffed taco; feel free to play with him for awhile if you would like! He'd also enjoy a short walk around the back yard on his leash.
WHO CAN DO THIS FOR ME?: My husband, my mother, my best friend, my neighbor.

TASK:

THINGS TO KNOW:

WHO CAN DO THIS FOR ME?:
_____

TASK:

THINGS TO KNOW:

WHO CAN DO THIS FOR ME?:
_____

TASK:

THINGS TO KNOW:

WHO CAN DO THIS FOR ME?:
_____

TASK:

THINGS TO KNOW:

WHO CAN DO THIS FOR ME?:
_____

TASK:

THINGS TO KNOW:

WHO CAN DO THIS FOR ME?:
_____

TASK:

THINGS TO KNOW:

WHO CAN DO THIS FOR ME?:
_____

TASK:

THINGS TO KNOW:

WHO CAN DO THIS FOR ME?:
_____

TASK:

THINGS TO KNOW:

WHO CAN DO THIS FOR ME?:
_____

TASK:

THINGS TO KNOW:

WHO CAN DO THIS FOR ME?:
_____

TASK:

THINGS TO KNOW:

WHO CAN DO THIS FOR ME?:
_____

TASK:

THINGS TO KNOW:

WHO CAN DO THIS FOR ME?:
_____

TASK:

THINGS TO KNOW:

WHO CAN DO THIS FOR ME?:
_____

TASK:

THINGS TO KNOW:

WHO CAN DO THIS FOR ME?:
_____

TASK:

THINGS TO KNOW:

WHO CAN DO THIS FOR ME?:
_____

TASK:

THINGS TO KNOW:

WHO CAN DO THIS FOR ME?:
_____

TASK:

THINGS TO KNOW:

WHO CAN DO THIS FOR ME?:
_____

TASK:

THINGS TO KNOW:

WHO CAN DO THIS FOR ME?:
_____

TASK:

THINGS TO KNOW:

WHO CAN DO THIS FOR ME?:
_____

TASK:

THINGS TO KNOW:

WHO CAN DO THIS FOR ME?:
_____

TASK:

THINGS TO KNOW:

WHO CAN DO THIS FOR ME?:
_____

TASK:

THINGS TO KNOW:

WHO CAN DO THIS FOR ME?:
_____

TASK:

THINGS TO KNOW:

WHO CAN DO THIS FOR ME?:
_____

TIP: *It may be helpful to use this same process when preparing to leave your job for an extended time. Fill in information for each of these questions as they pertain to your job duties, and share with your manager.*

surgery days

Use this space to think through the schedule of surgery days and what you might need.

DATE:_____TIME:_____HOSPITAL ADDRESS:_____

_____

WHAT TO PACK
- This journal!
- Loose-fitting, waistband-free clothing to wear to and from the hospital
- Shoes that are easy to put on and take off
- Small pillow to hold over your abdomen when you move, cough, sneeze, etc.
- Face wipes, lip balm, water bottle
- Encouraging cards or notes you may have received. These are great fear-fighters to read while you wait to be called into surgery.

caregiver information:

You will need someone to be with you at the hospital, to drive you home, and to stay with you for at least the first two days and nights that you are home.

WHO IS YOUR CAREGIVER?:_____

PHONE NUMBER:_____EMAIL:_____

AT-HOME CAREGIVER TASKS:
- Make sure you're resting and staying still
- Help you walk to the bathroom and get out of bed safely. Assist with catheter if you have one.
- Set alarms for your pain medications and make sure you take them on time (Stay ahead of the pain! Don't miss a dose.)
- Be sure you're drinking water regularly and refill your beverages as needed
- Answer the phone or door if you have visitors or meal or deliveries
- If you have kids at home, the caregiver should keep them busy and out of your resting area
- Offer you small amounts of food throughout the day
- Bring you ice packs, heating pads, or extra pillows as needed
- Make social media posts about your status after surgery if friends have requested that.

treatment days

Use this space to think through the schedule of treatment days and what you might need.

DATE:_____TIME:_____HOSPITAL ADDRESS:_____

_____

WHAT TO PACK
- This journal!
- Comfortable clothing to change into just in case you need to
- Warm socks, a hat, and a blanket
- Socks or slippers with gripped bottoms
- Entertainment to pass the time (books, tv shows, movies, puzzles, games)
- Face wipes, lip balm, water bottle
- Encouraging cards or notes you may have received.

caregiver information:

You will want to arrange rides to and from treatment. If you prefer to be alone during treatment sessions, have someone stay with you at home afterward for the rest of the day and possibly the next day, depending on how you tolerate treatment.

WHO IS YOUR CAREGIVER?:_____

PHONE NUMBER:_____EMAIL:_____

AT-HOME CAREGIVER TASKS:
- Make sure you're resting and undisturbed
- Help you get to the bathroom if you're weak
- Set alarms for any medications and make sure you take them on time
- Be sure you're drinking water regularly and not getting dehydrated
- Answer the phone or door
- If you have kids at home, the caregiver should keep them busy and out of your resting area
- Offer you small amounts of food throughout the day
- Help you manage your symptoms and stay comfortable

surgery days

Use this space to think through the schedule of surgery days and what you might need.

DATE:_____TIME:_____HOSPITAL ADDRESS:_____

_____

WHAT TO PACK
- This journal!
- Loose-fitting, waistband-free clothing to wear to and from the hospital
- Shoes that are easy to put on and take off
- Small pillow to hold over your abdomen when you move, cough, sneeze, etc.
- Face wipes, lip balm, water bottle
- Encouraging cards or notes you may have received. These are great fear-fighters to read while you wait to be called into surgery.

caregiver information:

You will need someone to be with you at the hospital, to drive you home, and to stay with you for at least the first two days and nights that you are home.

WHO IS YOUR CAREGIVER?:_____

PHONE NUMBER:_____EMAIL:_____

AT-HOME CAREGIVER TASKS:
- Make sure you're resting and staying still
- Help you walk to the bathroom and get out of bed safely. Assist with catheter if you have one.
- Set alarms for your pain medications and make sure you take them on time (Stay ahead of the pain! Don't miss a dose.)
- Be sure you're drinking water regularly and refill your beverages as needed
- Answer the phone or door if you have visitors or meal or deliveries
- If you have kids at home, the caregiver should keep them busy and out of your resting area
- Offer you small amounts of food throughout the day
- Bring you ice packs, heating pads, or extra pillows as needed
- Make social media posts about your status after surgery if friends have requested that.

treatment days

Use this space to think through the schedule of treatment days and what you might need.

DATE:_____ TIME:_____ HOSPITAL ADDRESS:_____

_____

WHAT TO PACK
- This journal!
- Comfortable clothing to change into just in case you need to
- Warm socks, a hat, and a blanket
- Socks or slippers with gripped bottoms
- Entertainment to pass the time (books, tv shows, movies, puzzles, games)
- Face wipes, lip balm, water bottle
- Encouraging cards or notes you may have received.

caregiver information:

You will want to arrange rides to and from treatment. If you prefer to be alone during treatment sessions, have someone stay with you at home afterward for the rest of the day and possibly the next day, depending on how you tolerate treatment.

WHO IS YOUR CAREGIVER?:_____

PHONE NUMBER:_____ EMAIL:_____

AT-HOME CAREGIVER TASKS:
- Make sure you're resting and undisturbed
- Help you get to the bathroom if you're weak
- Set alarms for any medications and make sure you take them on time
- Be sure you're drinking water regularly and not getting dehydrated
- Answer the phone or door
- If you have kids at home, the caregiver should keep them busy and out of your resting area
- Offer you small amounts of food throughout the day
- Help you manage your symptoms and stay comfortable

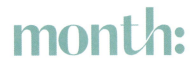

sun	mon	tues	wed	thurs	fri	sat

Use these calendars to organize and schedule helpers for your surgery and/or treatment days.

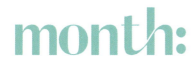

sun mon tues wed thurs fri sat

Use these calendars to organize and schedule helpers for your surgery and/or treatment days.

month:

sun	mon	tues	wed	thurs	fri	sat

Use these calendars to organize and schedule helpers for your surgery and/or treatment days.

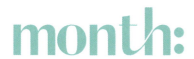

sun   mon   tues   wed   thurs   fri   sat

Use these calendars to organize and schedule helpers for your surgery and/or treatment days.

month:

sun	mon	tues	wed	thurs	fri	sat

Use these calendars to organize and schedule helpers for your surgery and/or treatment days.

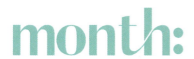

sun	mon	tues	wed	thurs	fri	sat

Use these calendars to organize and schedule helpers for your surgery and/or treatment days.

month:

sun	mon	tues	wed	thurs	fri	sat

Use these calendars to organize and schedule helpers for your surgery and/or treatment days.

month:

sun	mon	tues	wed	thurs	fri	sat

Use these calendars to organize and schedule helpers for your surgery and/or treatment days.

month:

sun	mon	tues	wed	thurs	fri	sat

Use these calendars to organize and schedule helpers for your surgery and/or treatment days.

month:

sun	mon	tues	wed	thurs	fri	sat

Use these calendars to organize and schedule helpers for your surgery and/or treatment days.

month:

sun	mon	tues	wed	thurs	fri	sat

Use these calendars to organize and schedule helpers for your surgery and/or treatment days.

month:

sun	mon	tues	wed	thurs	fri	sat

Use these calendars to organize and schedule helpers for your surgery and/or treatment days.

medication tracker

Show this section to your caregiver and ask them to write down each time you take medication. This will help you be sure you're staying on schedule and don't miss a dose.

Med:			Dose:			Time:

Med:			Dose:			Time:

Med:			Dose:			Time:

Med:			Dose:			Time:

Med:			Dose:			Time:

Med:			Dose:			Time:

Med:			Dose:			Time:

Med:			Dose:			Time:

Med:			Dose:			Time:

Med:			Dose:			Time:

Med:			Dose:			Time:

Med:			Dose:			Time:

Med: Dose: Time:

Med: Dose: Time:

Med: Dose: Time:

Med: Dose: Time:

Med: Dose: Time:

Med: Dose: Time:

Med: Dose: Time:

Med: Dose: Time:

Med: Dose: Time:

Med: Dose: Time:

Med: Dose: Time:

Med: Dose: Time:

Med: Dose: Time:

Med: Dose: Time:

Med: Dose: Time:

Med: Dose: Time:

Med:					Dose:					Time:

Med:					Dose:					Time:

Med:					Dose:					Time:

Med:					Dose:					Time:

Med:					Dose:					Time:

Med:					Dose:					Time:

Med:					Dose:					Time:

Med:					Dose:					Time:

Med:					Dose:					Time:

Med:					Dose:					Time:

Med:					Dose:					Time:

Med:					Dose:					Time:

Med:					Dose:					Time:

Med:					Dose:					Time:

Med:					Dose:					Time:

Med:					Dose:					Time:

Med:	Dose:	Time:
Med:	Dose:	Time:
Med:	Dose:	Time:
Med:	Dose:	Time:
Med:	Dose:	Time:
Med:	Dose:	Time:
Med:	Dose:	Time:
Med:	Dose:	Time:
Med:	Dose:	Time:
Med:	Dose:	Time:
Med:	Dose:	Time:
Med:	Dose:	Time:
Med:	Dose:	Time:
Med:	Dose:	Time:
Med:	Dose:	Time:
Med:	Dose:	Time:

Med:	Dose:	Time:
Med:	Dose:	Time:
Med:	Dose:	Time:
Med:	Dose:	Time:
Med:	Dose:	Time:
Med:	Dose:	Time:
Med:	Dose:	Time:
Med:	Dose:	Time:
Med:	Dose:	Time:
Med:	Dose:	Time:
Med:	Dose:	Time:
Med:	Dose:	Time:
Med:	Dose:	Time:
Med:	Dose:	Time:
Med:	Dose:	Time:
Med:	Dose:	Time:

Med: Dose: Time:

Med: Dose: Time:

Med: Dose: Time:

Med: Dose: Time:

Med: Dose: Time:

Med: Dose: Time:

Med: Dose: Time:

Med: Dose: Time:

Med: Dose: Time:

Med: Dose: Time:

Med: Dose: Time:

Med: Dose: Time:

Med: Dose: Time:

Med: Dose: Time:

Med: Dose: Time:

shop & stock up

For many women, the weekly task of picking up groceries, toiletries, and household supplies is built right into our schedule. We fit it into our lunch breaks and between dropping the kids off at school and sports. Use this space to think through what you might need to stock up on for yourself and/or your family before you begin treatment or surgery.

You might be advised not to drive or lift heavy bags for a little while after surgery, and anesthesia and pain medication may have you fighting some brain fog. Chemo and radiation may steal your strength and make it hard for you to run errands like you normally do. Your routine will be thrown off, to be sure. Having these items bought in bulk or just in advance will save you a lot of stress and worry going into your treatment or recovery time.

Add to the list on the next few pages, thinking through the staple items for you and your household. Make this list work for you. Let's start with the stuff you usually buy. I've gotten you started below.

household items

- paper products (paper towels, toilet paper, facial tissues)
- soaps (hand soap, dish soap, laundry detergent)
- cleaning products
- trash bags
- extra food storage bags/containers

personal items

- toothpaste/toothbrush
- OTC medications/prescriptions
- shampoo/body wash
- hair products
- lotion
- deodorant
- lip balm
- face wash

shop & stock up

Use this open space to jot down items as they come to you.

comfort & care supplies

Now let's shift our focus to what *you* need.
Many women only think about what those around them will need while they're going through treatment and/or surgery. Please hear me when I say the following:

Self-care is as crucial to cancer treatment and recovery as medicine.

There's one bit of criteria for this list: All of these items should be helpful and comforting. I've shared items below that I used often in my own cancer treatment experience. I also polled a group of other cervical cancer survivors who shared about their favorite things that helped and comforted them through their treatment. Some of these items have a medical purpose, like nausea-fighting ginger chews, ice packs, maxi pads and belly-support pillows. While others are just small ways to brighten your day when you're feeling low. Think fancy hand creams, scented body spray, extra bed pillows, a brightly-colored super-soft hat!

grocery items

- **crackers**
- **applesauce pouches** (unlike jarred or cup applesauce, they are shelf-stable and don't need to be refrigerated, so you can bring them with you or keep them bedside.)
- **bananas**
- **clean beverages** (water, caffeine-free tea, sparkling flavored water, etc.)
- **ginger chews or lozenges**
- **popsicles**

personal items

- **face wipes**
- **deodorant**
- **lip balm**
- **hand cream**
- **scented body spray**
- **dry shampoo**
- **hair ties or a hat**
- **sheet facial masks or undereye pads**
- **foot masks/peels**
- **scented candles**
- **a fun phone case** (you'll likely be spending a lot of time with your phone!)
- **ginger and/or lavender essential oil inhalers** (lavender helps calm anxiety and ginger helps reduce nausea)

surgery recovery items

- **small belly-support pillow**
- **loose loungewear** (avoid waistbands for the first few days)
- **cooling bedsheets** (search for moisture-wicking blends)
- **extra pillows** to lean on and arrange in bed and in your recovery space at home
- **hair ties, head scarves, or soft hats**— whatever makes you most comfortable!
- **water bottle/tumbler**
- **ice pack**
- **heating pad**
- **maxi pads**
- **soft cotton underwear** (one size larger than your normal size)

chemo/radiation items

- **Aquaphor®** for radiation side effects
- **comfortable clothing and soft blankets**
- **hair ties, head scarves, or soft hats**— whatever makes you most comfortable!
- **socks or slippers with gripped bottoms**
- **bucket with a lid and handle**, lined with a plastic bag for easy disposal
- **Immodium® and Preparation H®**
- **water bottle/tumbler**
- **ice pack**
- **protein-rich chemo-safe powders, drinks, bars**
- **coloring books and pencils/markers**

comfort & care supplies

Use this space to brainstorm about some things you'd like to have with you as you endure and recover from treatment. Create a shopping list, or start compiling an Amazon Wishlist to share with anyone who asks, "What do you need?"

mantras

- I will rest my body every single day.
- I will not lift anything heavier than recommended by my doctor sooner than I should. I will ask for help whenever I need it.
- I will adjust my expectations about what a clean home needs to look like.
- I will be kind to myself about my appearance.
- I will take naps if I feel tired. No shame.
- I will remember to take short walks at a reasonable pace each day.
- I will be open to seeking out counseling and/or mental health resources.
- I will take pain medication as needed and not try to tough it out.
- I will not shame myself for lack of productivity or daily accomplishments.
- I will accept and love my body as it is and not wish it looked different.
- I will call my doctor's office without delay with any worries as they arise.
- I will not rush recovery.

after treatment

The majority of treatments for cervical cancer cause permanent loss of fertility. There are some fertility-sparing approaches, but not everyone is eligible. Fertility becomes a heavy issue for many of us.

It's possible that you have children and are done with that chapter of your life. Saying goodbye to your reproductive organs may not feel like a very big deal to you. It's also possible you never wanted to be pregnant and are glad to see your monthly period go away. It's possible that you weren't sure if you wanted to be pregnant someday or not, but a cervical cancer diagnosis forced you to have to decide more quickly than you were ready to. No matter where your head and heart were before this diagnosis and treatment, your emotions will do what they want to do when you're going through it. It might hit you the minute you wake up from surgery as it did me. It might dawn on you like a pile of bricks in your gut, mid-infusion in the chemo lab.

It might hit you 6 months from now when your totally normal trip to the store for paper towels deteriorates into you running from the baby clothes section because your heart hurts too much to even look at those tiny overalls and sweater cardigans. (If this is you, head right over to the ice cream aisle. You deserve a pint.)

It might affect you every single day for months on end. Or you might wake up one morning with a smile on your face and feel sweet, sweet freedom and peace because you no longer have cancer and that's enough.

No matter how you look at it, this is a huge thing. Walking through this experience is not for the faint of heart. It takes strength and resilience and honesty and humility and vulnerability and a willingness to seek help and support. We cannot do it alone.

It is vital that you continue to tend to your emotional health after treatment. Check in with yourself. Ask yourself what you need. Don't expect too much from yourself. Write. Pray. Cry. Laugh with a friend (but don't forget to hold that pillow over your abdomen, first!). Grieve if you need to. Rejoice if you want to. Just don't act like nothing happened. Honor your experience.

March 10, 2019 // 11:15am

When I started to wake up in the recovery area after my hysterectomy, a kind nurse was waving a ginger essential oil inhaler in front of my nose and gently stroking my shoulder with her hand. I immediately started to cry.

The drugs wearing off, the tension releasing from months of fearing that day, an intense desire to be anywhere but there at that moment,

the overwhelming tender kindness she was showing me at one of the lowest points in my life, and realizing that I was now living in the reality of my female body without a cervix, uterus or fallopian tubes, all swirled together into a tornado of emotion. It was done. It really happened.

I dozed off and woke back up a million more times that day, both in the hospital and at home later that afternoon, and each time I would go through the same emotional cycle. Awaken, realize I officially can never be pregnant, my organs are gone, worry about lab results, cry a little, fall back asleep. The drugs helped me forget but I would just remember all over again a few hours later as if it was the first time.

time to process

How did you feel in the moments, hours, and days after surgery or when you ended treatment? How did you cope?

What emotions did you experience?

What has been the hardest thing about this season? What has been a bright spot throughout it?

after treatment

Use these pages to reflect and process through your experience of wrapping up treatment or beginning your recovery period. Think about moments you want to remember and what you'd rather forget. Write about it all openly and honestly here.

the wait

It's long. It's quiet. It's the worst.
You'll often hear cancer patients talk about The Wait as the worst part of their treatment experience. The anticipation and fear leading up to surgery or your first chemo day is one thing; but the experience of having a scan or a biopsy or a surgical operation, recovering mentally and emotionally from that, while simultaneously waiting to hear if the chemo is working, or if the cancer is back, worse, or completely gone is a whole other terrible thing. Here are some things you can do to help yourself through.

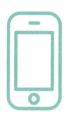
support
Make a list of friends and family you can call just to talk. It doesn't even have to be about cancer. Sometimes it's just nice to be distracted from the heaviness.

counseling
If you don't already see a professional counselor, ask your oncologist for a recommendation. You may even have a friend or family member who can recommend someone that you could talk to when you're feeling anxious or low.

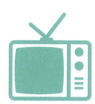
movies + tv
Make a list of movies and TV shows you'd like to watch while recovering. I found it very comforting to watch old shows that I used to enjoy when I was younger. Ask friends, family and social media for recommendations, too.

books
Make a list of books you'd like to read while recovering. I personally found it hard to push through brain fog from anesthesia enough to read while recovering, but I appreciated having another option for something to do besides watching TV. Even if I only read a few pages at a time, it felt good to use my brain. Ask friends, family and social media for recommendations and start reserving books at the library in advance. Many libraries also have audiobook apps.

music
Make uplifting, relaxing, or spiritually encouraging playlists or mix CDs to listen to while recovering. Sometimes it can feel good to just put headphones on and be transported somewhere else. Coloring, journaling, and working on puzzles are great activities to do while listening to music.

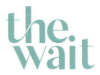
the wait

Use this space to jot down some ideas for ways that you can prepare to occupy yourself during The Wait.

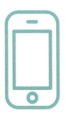
support

Who can you call or ask to visit you?

counseling

Write down the name, number, and/or website of a nearby counselor that you are willing to see once you're able. If you've been given instructions not to drive while you're recovering, consider asking a friend or family member for a ride. You may also consider temporarily utilizing one of several popular therapy apps available right on your phone.

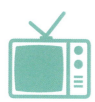
movies + tv
What do you want to watch? Write down which streaming services each show or movie is available on so they're easy to locate, either by you or your caregiver.

books
What do you want to read? Make a list of magazines or books you'd like to purchase or check out in advance. These are also great things to suggest if anyone asks what you need or what they can buy for you.

music
What do you want to listen to? Make a list of artists/musicians you find uplifting, soothing, or calming.

grief & gratefulness

From survivor's guilt to learning it's not over yet; Whatever your outcome, you may experience a multitude of emotions. In the same way that nothing prepares you for that phone call telling you that you have cancer, nothing can prepare you for what you find out after treatment. I'm here to tell you that you'll be swept up into a feelings tornado and the best thing you can do is let yourself feel it all. Don't try to stop it. Don't tell yourself you should feel any certain way. Feel your feelings. This is many things. It's both happy and sad, ugly and beautiful, darkness and light.

I remember a specific time that my grief got the best of me. While I walked through cancer and all of the unfairness that comes with it, my mom was understandably upset and hurting and wanted to help me however she could. I'm not proud of it, but I unleashed all of my feelings at her on the phone one day. I spewed anger and I yelled and I cried and I was unkind and I tried to push her away. Because she's my mom, and only because she's my mom, she absorbed all of it and didn't try to hurt me back. And she didn't walk away because of it, either. Those explosive emotions were 100% normal and 100% allowed. However, the way I handled them was not great. But my hope for you is that there's someone close to you who loves you and understands that you're going through something terrible, and you're not fully in control of your behavior. Grace is a gift and we need a lot of it every single day as we face the evils of cancer.

The complicated and intense emotions continued when I got my NED call. My mom was sitting with me at my apartment. I was still swollen from surgery, exhausted and a little foggy from anesthesia, when the nurse on the phone said they got it all, no chemo or radiation was needed, and I was cancer-free. She ended by cheerfully saying, "So you don't have to worry anymore!" I got the feeling I wasn't reacting the way she thought a person should after learning they were cancer free. I think I just flatly said, "Ok that's great news. Thank you."

My mom burst into tears of relief and hugged me. She was overjoyed. I was too. But all I could do was sit there on the couch, stare at the rug with my eyes welling up with hot tears, feeling empty inside. It was over. It was finally over. My mom said, "Aren't you happy?" Why didn't I feel happier? Because although I was cancer free and I got to move on with my life, I immediately thought of the women in my Cervivor™ support group who were still fighting. Those who'd lost their lives. It isn't fair.

I was also still coming to terms with the loss of my womb and any chance for my husband and I to have biological children. Sure, we could rejoice that I didn't have cancer anymore. But our lives were changed forever. And we lost a lot. There was a lot to grieve alongside our joy.

So if you find yourself conflicted or overwhelmed by your feelings, no matter your prognosis, remember that your feelings are allowed and valid. All of them. Happy and sad, relieved and grieved, shell-shocked but ready to move forward. The dark feelings come right alongside the light ones. There isn't any one way you're supposed to feel. Feel it all.

Use the next few pages to do some internal healing. Think about what you've lost through this experience. Write. Draw pictures. Make lists. Be honest and raw. Then, think about what you're grateful for in this moment. Consider what you've gained through this experience. Think about what cancer hasn't been able to steal from you. Revisit these pages when you need a tangible reminder that

things are never so dark that the light can't get in.

grief & gratefulness

what I'm grieving

grief & gratefulness

what I'm grateful for

the new normal

Look, I know that you just want to get back to your "normal life". But there's something you need to know—your life will never be the kind of normal it was before cancer. I didn't fully realize this until I was months past my treatment.

As surgery approached and I wrote in my journal, I worried about what life would look like after cancer. There was really no way to prepare myself, as badly as I wanted to somehow ready myself for what was coming. Cancer changes us forever in good ways and in hard ways. So before you start busying yourself with tasks to pick up where you left off before cancer exploded your life into a million pieces, come to terms with the fact that you simply cannot pick up where you left off. This is a new beginning.

Take this recovery time to be gentle with yourself, truly and deeply find rest, and prepare for what's next. I hope some of the things I learned will help you along the way.

Februrary 12, 2019 // 2:30pm

I'm starting to carry this so heavily. It feels like a death. Like when they put me under for surgery I'm going to die and wake up someone else. I guess that doesn't have to be bad. Life changes us, inevitably. But it's a little sad. Okay, a lot sad. And hard.

December 10, 2019 // 7:40pm

When I told my counselor back then that I was worried I was going to wake up from my hysterectomy as an entirely different person, she told me that she saw that as an exciting and empowering opportunity. To rise up into something brand new and hopefully get to strip away the C word from my life and focus on new things.

What I've learned as I've lived into my new post-cancer normal is that nothing is truly post-cancer. Cancer may not be in my body right now and hopefully never will be again, but it's in everything in my life and it always will be. It has changed me, my marriage, my future, my body, my mind. I've also realized that it isn't necessarily bad that these things have changed. They're just new and different.

I joined an online group of survivors of various cancers who are trying to get in shape after treatment or surgery. I have been frustrated with my progress with exercise. I avoid working out because it feels different than it did before my hysterectomy. I've lost so much strength and I get little pelvic pains sometimes and I'm reminded of my reality, and then I get sad and just quit. I shared this in the group and a wise women said, "Nothing will ever be how it was before. Don't expect yourself to look or behave how you did before cancer. Release those expectations and *just start new.*" Just start new.

That's what this next chapter of life has to be about. Not about getting back to where I was, but acquainting myself with my new body, my new perspective and mindset, and being gentle with myself through it all. Taking tiny little steps toward brand new goals.

Some recent goals have been to face my fear of seeing a pelvic floor therapist to help treat some of the pain I still have. I learned it's from excessive scar tissue and if I'm consistent with appointments, it can be helped. Each appointment is a tiny victory and one more step into a brighter next chapter.

Another goal has been to see a marriage therapist with Justin. We went through hell and it's time to get honest about it. We've been going for a month now and I already feel closer to him and it has immensely helped our connection to gain alignment together as we go forward. At each appointment, we punch cancer in the face and take our life together back by starting fresh again and again. I'm also going back to my counselor to deal with some recurrent traumatic dreams I've had about different parts of my treatment. Soon I'll have tools to help myself through those scary memories when they flare up.

Nothing will ever be the same. But I'm grateful to get to just start new.

This is a list of some common things that many cervical cancer patients experience as they adjust to life after treatment. This list is not meant to scare you, but prepare you. Keep in mind that everyone is different and you should not expect to encounter all of these things.

- You may feel fatigued or tired more easily than before. Motivation to exercise may come slowly but it will return eventually.

- Your body may look or feel different. You may need to reacquaint yourself with parts of your body that changed during treatment.

- You may suffer from some brain fog or slow cognition for awhile. Cancer trauma and cancer treatment are both taxing on the brain. Go easy on yourself as you catch up to your coworkers and peers.

- Using the bathroom may be a different experience than before. Work with a pelvic floor therapist to address issues and alleviate any side effects.

- If you had lymph nodes removed as part of your treatment, you may experience lymphedema. Your doctor will guide you through managing these symptoms.

- You may have gained or lost weight. So what? Don't obsess. Go easy on yourself and focus on good nutrition and whole, healthy foods.

- Your priorities may shift. This isn't necessarily bad and is likely a good thing. Work with a counselor to address any concerns as you rebuild and strengthen relationships affected by your cancer.

- You may need to continue taking medication long term.

- If you have your ovaries removed or they are affected by treatment, you may enter surgical menopause. Speak with your doctor about managing any side effects.

- Many cancer patients, regardless of their diagnosis and/or treatment, will experience some symptoms of PTSD (Post-Traumatic Stress Disorder). Some hallmark signs include irritability, reactive responses, vivid dreams or flashbacks, and avoidance of reminders of the trauma. If you find that you're having trouble in any of these areas, reach out to a counselor or your oncologist as soon as possible.

ways to cope

There are some things you can do to help yourself be as mentally and physically empowered as possible as you settle into this new chapter of your life. Try some of these helpful coping strategies to set yourself up for a peaceful, supported return to regular day-to-day activities.

- **Sign up for a yoga or meditation class or look for free videos online.** Gentle yoga is a great way to go easy on your body while starting to engage in physical exercise again. Balance, core strength, and flexibility are focuses of these practices—three crucial components to healing from radiation, chemotherapy and surgery.
- **Reach out to a spiritual advisor.** Consider tapping into your spiritual side, if you have one. If you're a person of faith, connect with your house of worship or a friend with similar beliefs to your own. Discuss what you've been through and how your faith can play into your healing.
- **Buy a new journal.** I think it's really important to mark this new chapter as significant. Start fresh. Pick out a nice journal at your local bookstore or online and keep writing about your feelings and emotions. Continue processing whenever you feel overwhelmed or confused, or experience happy moments that you want to record and remember later. Starting a daily gratefulness journal is also helpful for many survivors.
- **Look for ways to give back.** Many cancer patients feel compelled to give back to the cancer community or their friends and family after treatment. After receiving support, we're often filled up and ready to pour out some of the kindness we've received. Look for volunteer opportunities at churches, schools, public libraries, community centers, senior centers, and cancer clinics.
- **Share your experience publicly, if you feel comfortable.** For many cervical cancer survivors, advocacy becomes important. Because there is so much misinformation about HPV and cervical cancer in our society, we feel empowered to correct the lies and educate our communities. Consider using your social media platforms to share your story and accurate, reputable news articles about HPV and cervical cancer from organizations like Cervivor™, the CDC and American Cancer Society.
- **Set expectations with family and friends**. Many of our family members and friends were traumatized by watching us face cancer and they may be anxious for you to fully return to being the person they knew before you were diagnosed. While that is understandable, they should not impose a timeline upon us for when we should be back to, "normal". If there's anyone in your life that voices concern that you're not, "back to normal", it may be helpful for them to speak with your oncology team. Your doctor(s) can explain that this is a holistic healing journey and it will take some time. You may also want to remind them that the normal they knew is gone, and you're now adjusting to a new way of life.

the new normal

Use this space to create a survivorship plan for yourself. Make tangible goals like setting appointments for checkups with your oncologist and/or primary care physician. Reach out to a mental health counselor. Ask for a pelvic floor therapist referral. Sign up for a yoga class. You get to decide what your life looks like going forward, regardless of your circumstances. Begin the framework for this next chapter of your life, here.

the new normal

the new normal

every thing is going to be Ok

(even if everything is the opposite of okay today.)

thank you

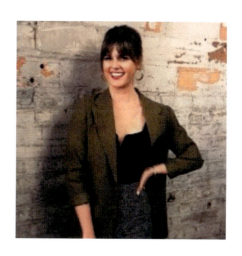

To my husband Justin. For more love, grace, understanding, and support in sickness and in health than I have words to thank you for. To family, friends, coworkers, and total strangers for love, care, and encouragement beyond my wildest, craziest dreams. To my friends, for encouraging me to find my lady guts and finish this project. To the Cervivor™ community and Facebook Group: where there's no question too graphic, no situation too silly, no story too sad and heavy to be carried by the incredible group of survivors there. I cherish their camaraderie. And to my longtime counselor/therapist, Amanda. Without you, I don't know how I could have ever coped with all that cervical cancer threw my way. I'm so grateful to be able to share some of what you taught me with other women who need it.

mostly, thank you.

Thank you for the honor of accompanying you through your cervical cancer journey.
Keep fighting. Keep educating. Keep advocating.
This cancer is preventable. Let's do everything we can to keep other women
from having to walk through what we've walked through.

I started this book by saying, "You are stronger than you know."
Through this, I hope you've come to know the depth of your strength.
Go forward and live in it.

*Andrea Bonhiver is a cervical cancer survivor living in Minneapolis, MN
with her husband Justin and their 11-year old Yorkie child, Louis.*

Made in the USA
Monee, IL
02 February 2020

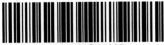